Health Information Benefits Fitness, Wellness, How To Diet, Eating, Care

Healthy Healing Living Habits For Women, Men, Children How To Benefit

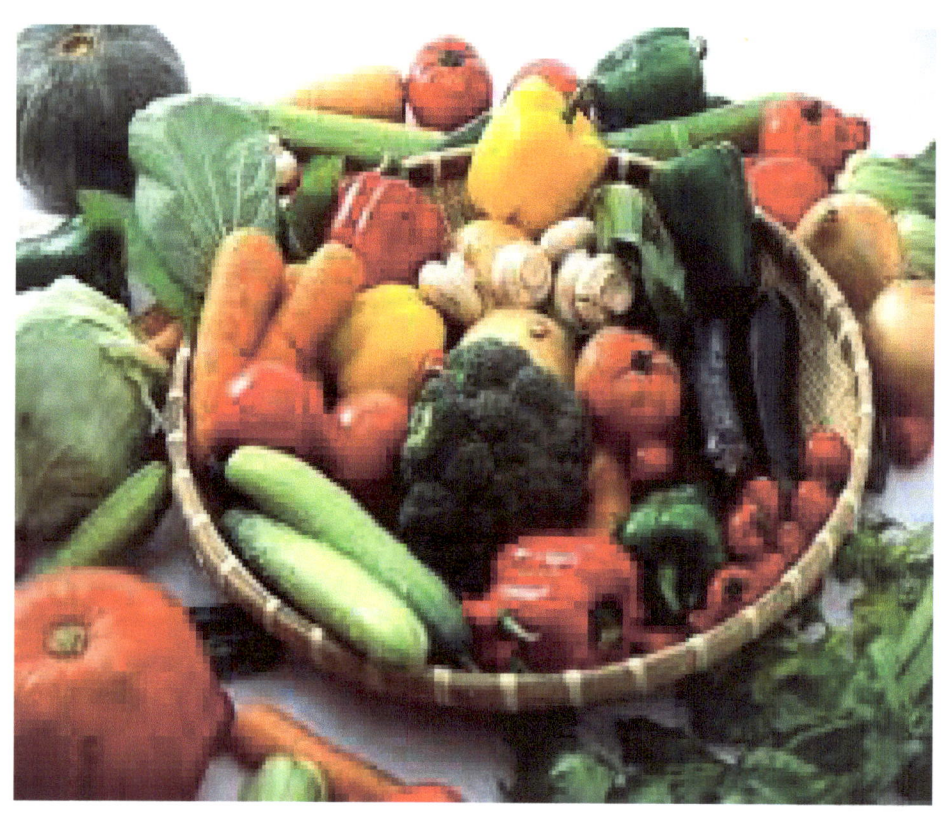

Table of contents

Chapter 1

Health is very important to us, in these times we have pesticides in all our foods and vegetables. Most of our citizens in America and people worldwide global suffer from health problems. We have fast food restaurants on almost every street corner. Burger king, Mc. Donald's, Wendy's, Taco bells etc; Also these fast foods are in growing populations of cities and countries. Like Asia, Africa, Puerto Rico, China. Misinformation has clouded our minds for big business manufacture companies, who make millions of dollars off people ignorance. We don't look very far to seek out information about a glitzy celebrity miraculously losing 40 lbs in ten days or a much loved public figure, succumbing to a terrible heart attack.

In the darkest hours, many people are so numb. The glossy covers of slim bodies are unreal also feeling the shock of those who are sickly, and barely hanging on make us look distance. What tabloids mean? What are they inadvertently trying to warn us or tell us! Ask? Perhaps we can take a few minutes to post at least two questions dealing with life. What is health? And why is it very important?

Health is very difficult and complex. We can focus on a few acute areas, Look at the human body. As we begin to work on our vessel as an overriding concept, our health relates to the heart capacity to pump blood in the internal organs the ability to absorb nutrients provided through food, water, and other intakes. The agility of our muscles, bones to twist and move, and of course cells working optimally to reproduce and repair when damaged. Don't forget the brain, spine, arteries, and all those micro-small neurotransmitters sending signals. So many wonderful surprising connections are happening in the human body at any given time. Let us give homage to it as one complete universal body that stands for health and it's essential.

Keeping our bodies in good condition benefits the individual health, without it we cease to function as productive members of society and as a member of the human race. If health should decline to the lowest levels one can become susceptible to obesity, diabetes, hypertension, also become vulnerable to a myriad of chronic diseases. With that being said, the choices we make can give us advantageous to long life and health to operate at peak standards. All the pieces interconnect for adequate health, choosing good food. Clean spring water is better than unhealthy water.

Exercising daily includes your mind and body. Each conscientious effort will begin transforming the human physical body into it's own personal accountability, toward safety prevention of food choices.

Chapter 2

Medical related needs, physical exertion and the rest begin with health. Instead of thinking with our stomach we need to control our mind which will in time bring balance in our life. Most people live their life in a program. Every day we watch these shows and our subconscious record them. It's just a matter of time that we will exercise those thoughts into reality and feed our physical body the wrong diet. When you are in the supermarket read the labels, check for everything sodium is one of the reasons for high blood pressure and other health related issues. Salt will kill you, too much of it may. White sugar is very bad for our body intake. Use brown sugar it's better, Most sugary foods like cake, cookies, muffins, donuts, and the list goes on let's not forget candy which in time destroy our teeth and body with diabetes. Our ignorance of not being responsible for our thoughts display through the action of the body functioning process. Too much of anything can cause the wrong turn sending us to the doctor making him or her rich. Rice, potatoes, starches in general.

Cardiac arrest is very high all over the world. Too much of butter, oil, grease of any kind, builds up in the arteries, clogging the arteries to the point where the blood gets jam from the natural flow. It's like a beaver building a dam. The beaver make sure most of the water doesn't go through the other side, making sure the home is secure. You can learn a lot from animals.

Strokes are at a high percentage. Most strokes come from a condition of the brain cells which suddenly die. The reason is lack of oxygen which in fact can cause an obstruction in the blood flow. Some of the reasons that can cause these health problems are poor diet, smoking, high levels of bad cholesterol, also stress which we all go through at times. Another is when we're dealing with family, work, driving your car, going to school not having money to handle responsibilities. The list goes on and on. Try not to put a lot on your table, what I mean is when a situation occurs sit back and relax, things have its own way of working out. Don't crowd your thoughts with confusion. Let nature and time balance its way out. Some situations we don't have control over, matters which can be a learning example to grow in different ways of life.

Obesity comes from too much eating as well the wrong foods. Most of us eat all day and some of us eat five times a day. Not allowing the body time to process all the chemicals that's in pesticides. The work that we are putting on our organs and arteries are causing them to work harder and longer which we ignore. It's time to open our minds to the reality of health for our bodies. Nobody is going to take care of you better than your own self. How do you know when you're at obesity level? Look at your normal weight. Once you step on the scale and your weight is above 20% of your normal body weight you are in that class of obesity excessive proportion of total body fat.

Chapter 3

 Some people get upset when being told their 20 to 40 pounds overweight. Eating yourself to death is very dangerous. These calories are pushed to the side because the machine which is our body, is working on the next math problem we just digested. It takes at least 24 hours for the body to properly distribute food into proper areas where it needs to go.

The body is a vehicle, the engine is the heart the oil is the blood, Just like a car that needs oil change, we need a better cleaner mind frame toward what we put in our mouth it can keep us here alive, or take us away. It's your choice! You decide what you want for a better future with no one taking care of you when you become old age. Think about it. Knowledge supersedes ignorance at all times. Communication is the key. How can you communicate with yourself and get good results. When you plant a seed in the dirt, you make sure it's planted in the right soil as well you placed it in the correct spot so now the sun and heat can make it germinate with water. Our bodies need tender loving care. We can't live without clean spring water. We can't live without food that's properly produced and suitable to eat. The best food I recommend is organic. There for we don't have to deal with dangerous chemicals that are not good for the human body.

How to reduce hypertension? We must not apply to much pressure on the heart. You need to reduce your salt intake on your diet. Most of us really don't check the high sodium that's in all these products, rice already has sodium in the bag or box, so why apply more salt. Just look at the label. A salty meal with rice taste so good but in the long run it will start destroying your body system. The affect may come in days, months, years. Diabetes and high blood pressure is the enemy of self destruction, if not treated without any control and self discipline, you will definitely reap the consequences, you need to exercise daily at the gym.

Stop smoking cigarettes! Stop drinking alcohol without any limitations of control regulation of

rules! You know the warning the government put on the labels, but you ignore the warning because you think it feels good and at that time you don't feel the affect taking place but in due time it will start to work on you, starting from inside the body, you can't visualize it, then outside the body aging you and taking away your natural beauty. The same way we started these habits we must stop them. We can change them for the better of health.

Work on your survival it's simple. Just stop and read all the labels of food and drinks you buy. That will help you decide which better choices of products that will relax your thoughts and mind with better knowledge of things. These times we live in are very serious, always look for good solutions that will open up your life expectation of nutrition which will grow and elevate your life for absolutely great health. We don't want to keep on going to the doctor with the same old problems, we know better than that, manage and maintain your money in your pocket, then we will have more money to save, for bills, rent, light bill, internet, cable, water, heat etc.

Chapter 4

High Cholesterol is building up in our cell membranes causing the inner and outer layer to build up. It prevents hydrocarbons which work in the membranes not allowing the crystallization of the hydrocarbons. Some causes of this are excessive meat eating, cooking oil, butter that can cause coronary heart disease. Some foods taste so good but in return it destroys our physical and internal organs that have a job to do when we eat the wrong foods. When you are suffering from chest pains also shortness of breath or other body weakness, contractions and all types of body disabilities you need to take extra precautions about the food you eat. Exercise to decrease your weight. Start aligning yourself with the correct knowledge leading to a happier life. Information is the key and eye opener. Changing to purify your life style would be amazing to the body positively. Different fruit and vegetable diets will give us the satisfaction to be grateful towards the heavenly body. You will live longer and look younger.

Chapter 5

We should turn away from eating pork, beef and all red meats that contribute to bad health, and other illness that follow behind the destruction of our vessel functioning process. We shouldn't be trying to put a job in our body that it can't handle, eating food late and going to sleep after will over work the body. The body needs help from a conscious mind of elevation, and good health. We have all had a time in our life when someone, family members or friends told us we're eating the wrong food. Why when people hear the truth they don't listen to the warning, but when you start feeling the side effects reality kicks in. Your body is not functioning properly now you on your way to see a doctor, only if you would have listen to the truth from family members and friends, who studied the truth, dealing with cause and effect the doctors wouldn't have to prescribe deadly medications.

The reality of time in which we live every day not thinking of all the good things we have. Some of us have eyes to see and some of us are born blind without eye sight or lose them to different accidents and causes. Diabetes can take away your physical ability. Your eyes are part of that beautiful blessing. Being able to see great wonders and describing them in colors are amazing. The hands we work with, clean, drive, play sports with; basketball, football, baseball also become authors with. The list goes on! We must give a thought of a reality check to one's self mind and body. Appreciate the gift of life.

The power of thought that works in all our minds can change the process of bad habits. When we work on our conscious level it will advance the health motivation to ignore the white sugar, the bleach white bread, red meats, scavengers of the sea and ponds, Shrimps, Crabs, Catfish, Lobsters and so on.

We have to start taking steps to learn a better way to eat. It takes twenty four hour for our body to distribute impurities. These impurities need to exit the body. Don't allow them to stay inside the body. It causes health issues such as tumor diseases, bone diseases, obesity, strokes, clogged arteries etc.

Chapter 6

Being slim doesn't let you off the hook because some slim bodies aren't eating and exercising. The slim person can fall into the same health issues that cause the body to react differently to abnormal health. Most of my examples are basic teaching to open the eyes, of the individual to be aware of products on the shelf, and fast food restaurants.

Try to eat between 3 to 4 PM. Also eat at the same time again that will allow the body time to handle the pesticides and impurities that was just digested. Eat to live not live to eat. We have reversed the way we naturally think, eat, drink, walk, sit and sleep. It's time to stand up, focus on the truth which will keep us here on earth longer and make us happier and wiser.

Cooking your own food and being able to manage your food knowing what and how much to apply in the measurement cup or table spoon, will give you the advantage of not allowing other people to give you the wrong balance of diet. Using too much salt will take you to the hospital either fast or slow.

Chapter 7

Being mindful will make you strong and take you a long way ignoring to do for self will allow someone else to control your thoughts. Don't let the restaurants and food companies win your money.

Eat fresh foods and cook them from scratch, don't eat processed foods it will destroy your body. If you own land or have a backyard you can start working on a garden and grow your own vegetables, wheat, fruits. Clean vegetables are healthy good because your time and dedication help produce organic products, not commercial pesticides harmful to the biological physical body.

Most of us are living on a program. Dunkin Donuts makes a lot of money off all that sugar donuts that they sell every morning and evening. It's so hard to process all that sugar, we have candies in every store. Candy destroys your teeth as well the body. Corn syrup is almost in all the products in the supermarkets. No natural foods these markets are providing. Food lions, Big lots and Walmart. The manufactures are the ones who help feed us. Good health is going downhill and dangerous health is uprising.

These symbolic messages that we watch on TV, movies, videos, cell phones also in the movie theaters, as we are watching these symbolic messages. We start to think we need to have a drink of Coca cola or Pepsi the way the program works is your subconscious picks up the message and now you think you need to have some popcorn or a drink at the time. For example you're watching television and then a commercial comes on during the break of a movie or episode, you see the desert and the hot sun a man on a bicycle sweat coming down his face, he opens a bottle of Pepsi, as the heat makes the man sweat he continues to drink, which suppose to relieve him from the sun in the desert heat. Now you feel like you are thirsty you go out to the corner store or market looking for what you seen in the television, caught by the symbolic message. The same situation happens with the cereal commercials, we get caught by the symbolic message brand of cereals and now we go out and buy it. You don't even know that process cereals have corn syrup in it. Corn is not for humans to eat, it's for cattle.

I know it taste good but are we studying what goes in the body. Depreciating the body and not caring for a healthy system. Let the body break down the poisons and distribute it out and what's good and nutritious the body will keep in.

Most people watch the commercials with their children's soon as the child see the new pop-tarts, cup cakes, devil dogs a lot more the list goes on. Soon as the commercial finish. The children ask the parent or vise versa the parent might ask "would that be something you would like to eat".

Start educating your children to be healthy and eat more fibers, fruits nutritional goodies. Being conscious and aware will keep them in the world longer, and not pay the Doctor for the parent ignorance. Change is good and change will work. If you love your children educate them to a better life style of living, it will help them with their children in the long run.

Chapter 8

Our teeth are very important. The mouth can cause problems on the heart and nervous system. When the teeth get damaged it can cause many things to happen. Headaches, migraines, neck ache, sinus issues, teeth bleeding, neck swelling, chest infections and numerous colds. Basically your mouth is the gateway to all nasty germs that will accumulate into the body. You can run into lots of health issues more than you think. Leaving your mouth untreated can cause different things like gum diseases. Many people are exposed to Radiation not knowing the great danger of a microwave. People rather eat microwavable foods instead of home cooked meals. Try to cook your foods naturally. Yes we all know that microwave food will cook faster but take a little time out of your busy day to prepare a meal with a pot or put it in a pan for the oven. It's that simple, protect yourself. Let's not forget about the television we sit in front of most of the day or night. I would like to mention when people have illnesses they go to see a Doctor sometimes they will recommend an x-ray from the x-ray machine, the devices will emit radiation. The cell phones, laptops, too much energy at high frequency can affect new cells which are radioactive and remove useful cells. Too much is bad for the health. What can help will be navy beans. Boil the navy beans and after they are cook you can apply a little butter and Ms. Dash no salt herbs seasoning for flavor. This will cut down the radiation in the cells of the body. Make sure it is organic navy beans they are the best ones. Microwavable popcorn destroys you slowly. Radiation can activate cancer cells. It taste good but at the same time you're watching a movie and not watching your health. Second truth is microwavable popcorn bags are bad for you, more terrifying than watching a horror flick. Hidden dangers is package and coated with

Chemical that's linked to cancer. It's poison eating popcorn. Did you know that the popcorn bags are coated with the chemical called perfluorochemicals, which is connected to various cancers it will damage the reproductive system. We have to be knowledgeable about the packaging as well. I am giving you an eye opener to be aware of foods and drinks that can affect the body. This knowledge is for self and family, children and friends. Digestive diseases could be cause by genetically modified organism. These food ingredients haven't been tested long term towards people health.

Places to be aware of that consist of high sodium. High concentrated salt. Popeye's chicken tenders 2,120 mg sodium. Hardees 2/3 lb thick burger 2,770 mg sodium. Taco bell's volcano nachos 1,670 mg sodium. Most Chinese restaurants P.F Chang's beef and broccoli 3,752 mg sodium. Arby's breakfast sausage gravy biscuit 3,754 mg sodium. Dunkin donuts bagel 4,520 mg sodium. Papa john's cheese sticks 6,700 mg sodium. May I go on to inform you of more, there are thousands of places, supermarkets that sale you products like the one's mention above. Your health is in your hands avoid unhealthy dishes. You would have to eat lots of broccoli which has potassium in it to compensate the large amounts of salt digestion. Check potato chips, french fries, cornflakes, skim milk, Italian dressing, pretzel twists, pasta sauce, large glass of tomato juice.

Most readers that acknowledge the facts of advice in my book will improve their life as an individual towards better health choices of food and beverages. People live longer by respecting the proper life style of nutrition. I am going to give you life saving vegetables/fruit that will improve your health, open your mind put your money where it will prolong life with information that is useful mentally and physically. What we eat and drink is very important it determines our state of living. People have many diseases affecting them today, bad habits which are crucial to the health, making wrong decision has cause physical problems with tremendous health issues. The body needs the right nutrition, not fast food products. Research the foods understanding what's in the food how it affects the health. Make the right decision to avoid health issues.

Chapter 9

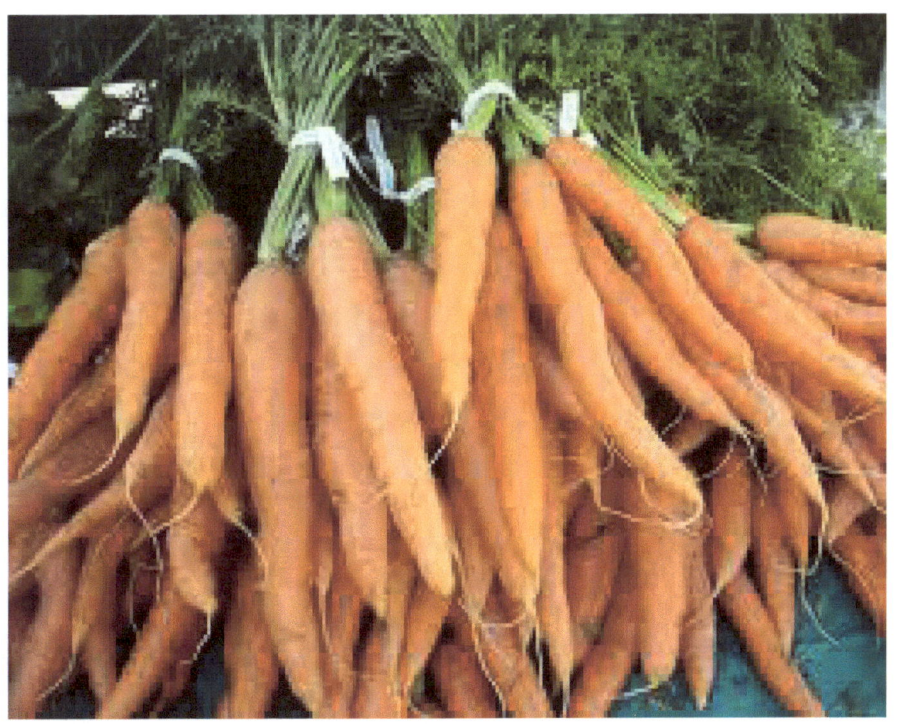

Carrots

Carrots and their properties are known for vitamin A they are a very precious vegetable. It has iron which is good for your blood and other things. Folic acid which helps the body make new cells healthy. Magnesium every part of the body needs this mineral kidneys need it, especially the muscles and the heart. Manganese, work on the bones building enzymes. Potassium helps with normal blood pressure. Carrots are your friend get to know them they will make a differents in your life. Our blood, digestive system, nervous system and the Integumentary system, depend on carrots to keep the balance of structure in the physical body. It's an excellent source with antioxidants that protect against lung cancer, and other types of health issues. Our immune system needs the right food to boost ailments by treating a range of poor cells. Also our stomach needs to be protected from ulcers.

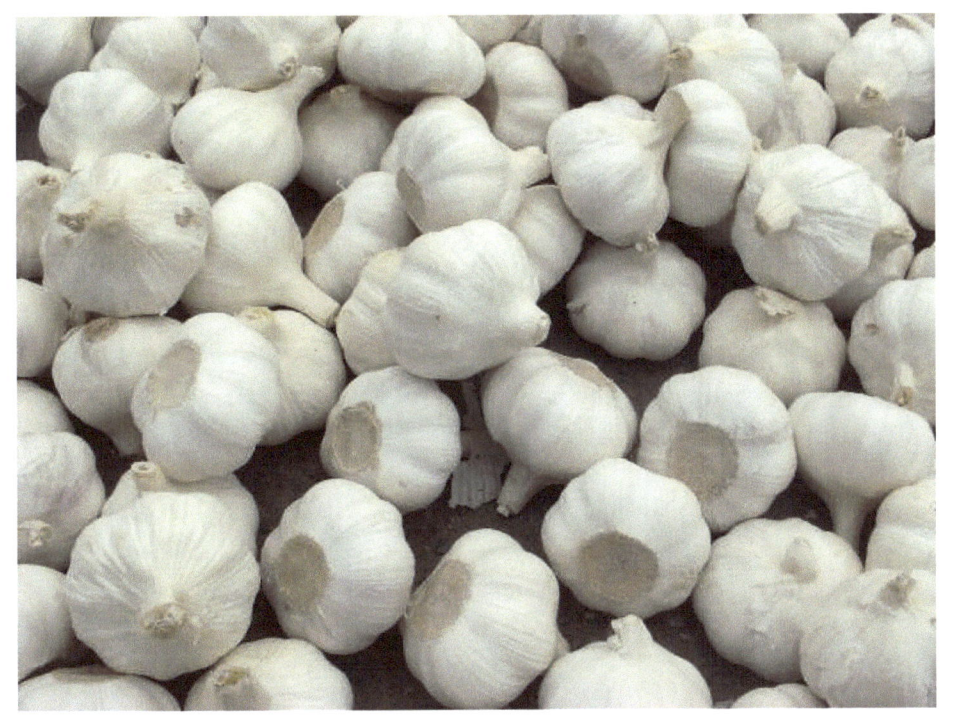

Garlic

Garlic is my favorite herb/vegetable. It protects and reduces cholesterol, anti-bacterial and Antifungal that works as a team in the system preventing illnesses. It works as a cure unblocking blood clots, also breaking down the buildup of existing clots. It helps reduce blood pressure, garlic also help the liver. It Suppresses production build up of cholesterol then it is expelled from our body. Raw garlic is the best, extremely useful remedy when you are sick. You can suck on a raw piece of garlic or chew on it instead, once it gets in your pores it start working magic. It's best to stay at home because most people can smell the garlic through the pores. Raw garlic relieves lots of symptoms like respiratory infections, nasal congestion, also heart diseases. I personally cook garlic in most of my foods. Sometimes I eat it raw it helps my system very well. Organic vegetable are good for you. Following these great steps will improve your circulatory problems which will make your organs smile.

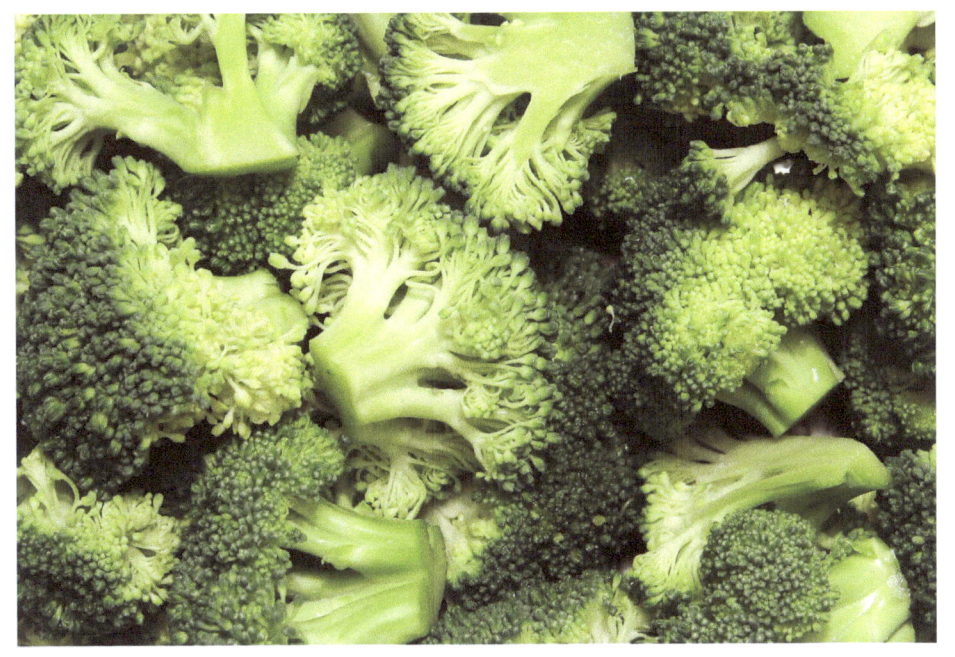

Broccoli

Broccoli has a great source of vitamin A and vitamin C it contains chromium, folic acid and calcium. These properties have been known to work against cancer. Broccoli sprouts are the root source of antioxidant which contains sulforaphane, glucosinolate.

The vitamin C can be used as a treatment to cure sinus infections. Sulforaphane has the ability to prevent bacteria that cause stomach ulcers. When you're out in the supermarket look for broccoli that's dark green color, make sure the heads on it are compact check for firm stalks. After buying, make sure you eat it in one or two days there for you get the greater extent of nutrition substance. These remedies have been around for a long time, eating raw broccoli will give you the best results that promote powerful abilities supporting and building bones, boosting the immune system, also it lower incidence of cataracts. The best way to cook broccoli is steaming the plant lightly.

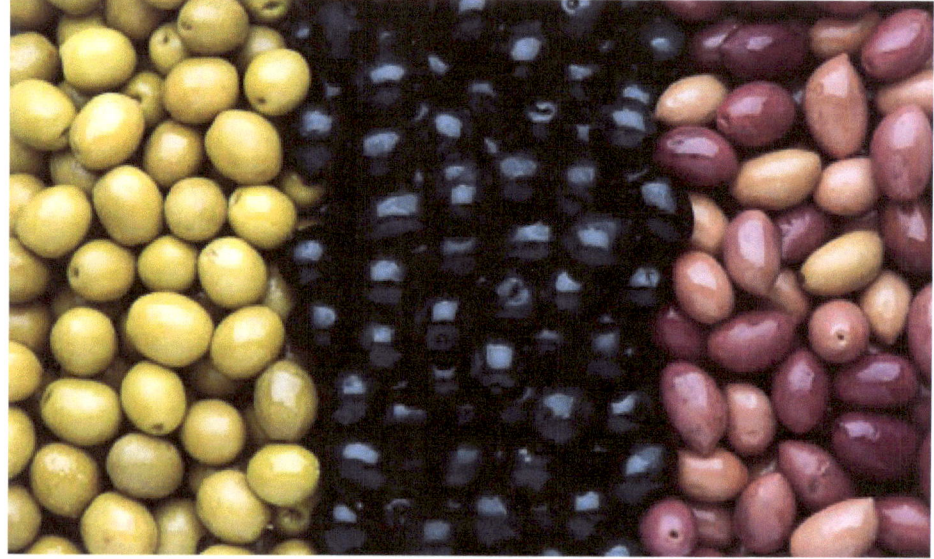

Olives

Olives are great for many things most restaurants use them in their magnificent serving dishes. Lots of people eat olives in there salads, some people cook olives in their rice, spaghetti, macaroni, bake toast or even pasta. Olive oil is obtained by the stone mill crushing the olives. New techniques have been used to extract the oil which superseded traditional ones. Virgin olive oil coloring may vary from different countries to another. It's a valuable fruit. Make sure you don't use semi fine as well refined olive oil. Olive produce vitamin A and vitamin E which can prevent particles being pass down arteries that produces different types of cardiovascular diseases. It can also help towards diabetes and gallstones. A lot of people use olive oil in their hair, on their skin it definitely helps with dry skin. Olive oil is also in shampoo and conditioner to strengthen and thicken the hair volume for fullness boost. Woman use it for nutrients for silky hair. Black olives work better on the digestive system, higher in vitamin level and antioxidant content other than green olives.

Chapter 10

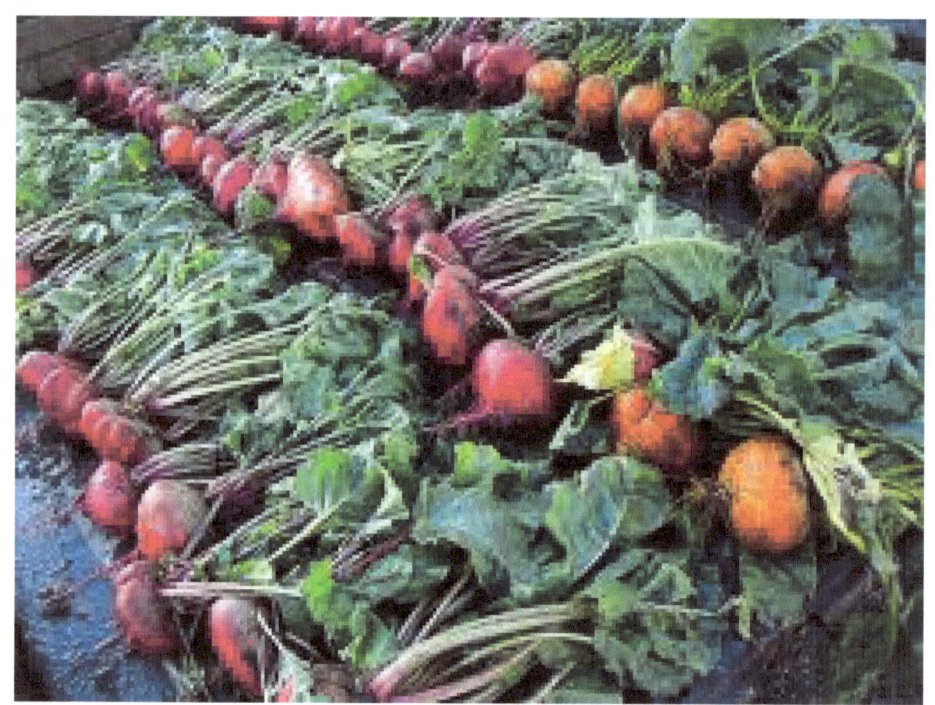

Beets

Beets are a powerful vegetable it has no harmful effects. It improves health and stimulates the immune system, effective treatment towards disorders in the blood. It aids in the immune system encourage production of the red blood cells also tissue oxygenation. Beets will aid the Respiration system towards muscles, nerves and the heart keeping them in excellent condition. Evidence has been proven that eating beets can push cancer cells to convert back to normal or just die. Beets have the ability to stabilize the body level by balancing acid alkaline. I like to eat beets raw because the natural minerals run through my immune system giving me energy for days, weeks and months. You can eat this vegetable with almost any dish. Beets have been used to treat leukemia, liver diseases, skin problems and inflammatory bowel disease. There are more solutions that the beets can help to restore normal body functions that were damage from poor eating habits. Maintaining a positive outlook on vegetables that can keep us here on earth, it's important that we take care of this human body or it will slowly bring us into different health issues that we will regret in our senior years or younger years. Beets help with mental health issues. It contains betaine, the same thing they use for certain treatments of depression. Beets are good for you so I suggest you start eating it daily because it reduces high blood pressure and it's a very excellent high source of energy.

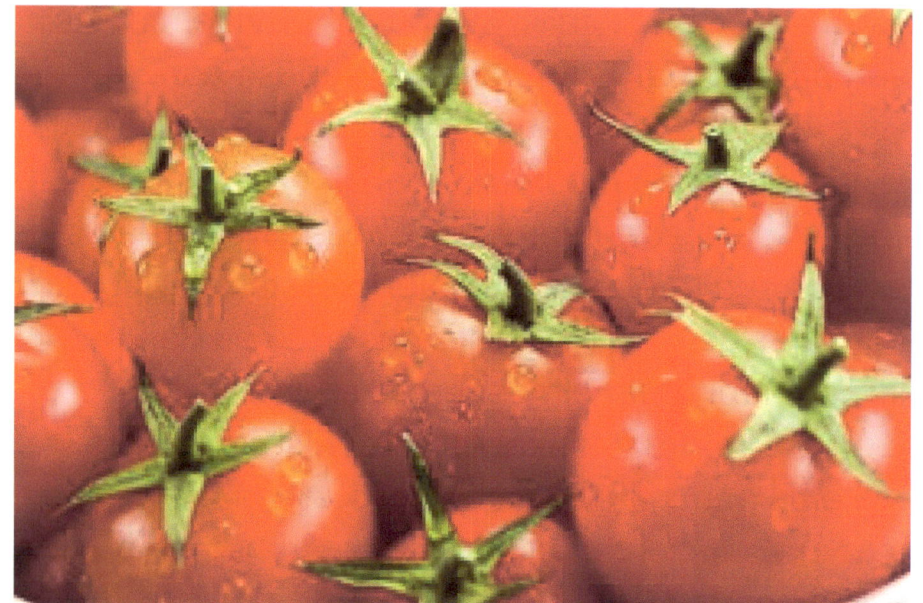

Tomatoes

Tomatoes are delicious an extremely wonderful vegetable/fruit. Most people use it in cooking meatballs, spaghetti, vegetable soup, salads, eggs, rice and beans.

Tomatoes are available all year around also relatively inexpensive. They are good for soups in the winter as well stews. Let's not forget pizza and ketchup. Tomatoes have the ability to reduce coronary artery disease, lung and skin problems as well stomach cancer. The pigment red color that is rich on the skin of the tomatoes is able to protect cells that are damage from oxygen damage. I try to eat raw tomatoes once a week they are very healthy for you. Lycopene is very valuable to many parts of the body structure fighting diseases in addition promoting important nutritional health. Vitamin C, vitamin B other benefits as well, you can grow this amazing vegetable in your backyard, in a large flower pot, hang it up in the back of the house or the front of the house. It's so simple to start a garden of your own.

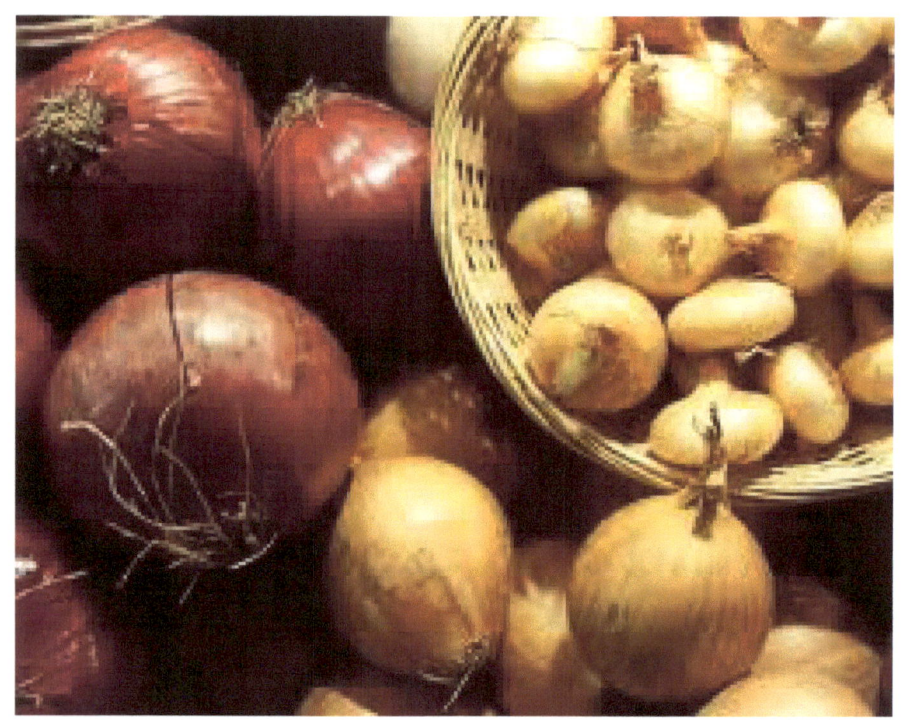

Onions

Onions produce properties of antifungal also antibiotic which has been known to reduce the levels in blood cholesterol it can also help with blood clots forming in the body. Onions have been useful in digestive plus circulatory system. Onions can be used for different issues, like colds or coughs, diarrhea that will keep you running to the bathroom day and night. They are an excellent vegetable that contains fiber and folate. Onions have been used for remedies in different parts of the world treating scars, as well as healing blisters, helping boils and working on damaged skin. They are rich in phytochemical, quercetin that can work against the effects of lung cancer, colon plus liver cancer. Onions make a great meal, you can eat it in many different ways, a lot of us apply them in soups, rice, burritos, chicken, beef and turkey. Eating onions raw is good for your health as well try to buy the organic ones. Fresh from the farm land, avoid canned onions avoid soft ones. Look to see if the skin is firm. Being healthy is the goal to living a long life without needing a home health aide in the long run.

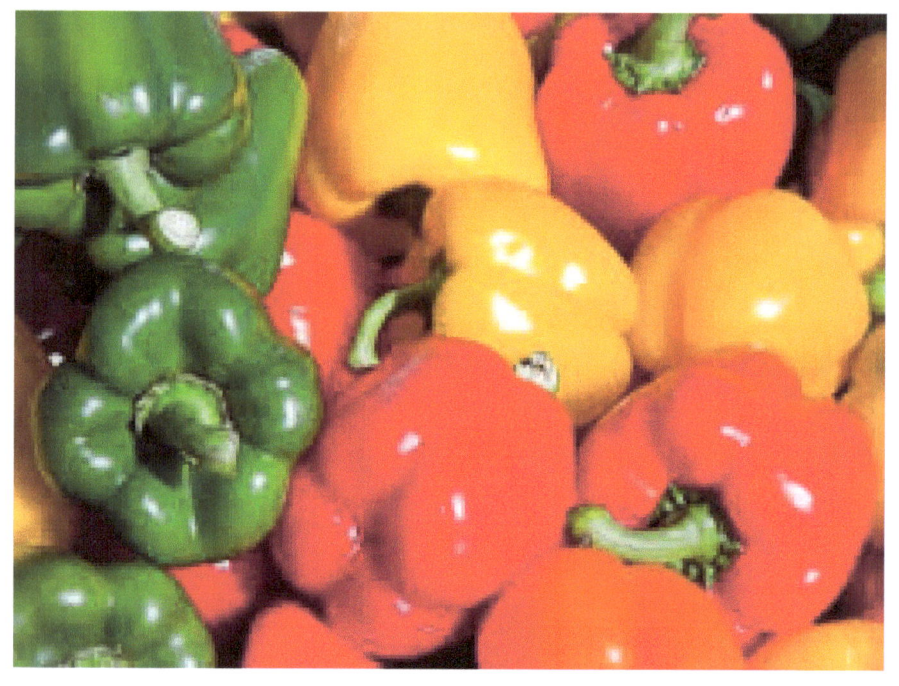

Peppers

Peppers come in different colors, green bell peppers and red peppers contain vitamin C and B. It has Flavonoids and anti-inflammatory effects that reduce phytochemicals. Each of the bell peppers differs with flavor plus heat intensity that has health nutrients, it benefits when you have a sore throat. Eating the pepper will relieve the inflammation building up in the system. Try eating natural vegetables to replenish the body system. Green, yellow, red and purple peppers are used in most of our home remedies. Most people in different countries like Mexico, India, Nigeria also other countries I didn't mention produce this vegetable as food and also healing purposes. The value of the pepper is needed and shown in most of the cooking chef's shows and restaurants. It has an excellent spicy taste and the Mexican people eat them in their burritos, tacos and beans. Make sure when you're going to the supermarket or the grocery store choose the right pepper the one with the tight skin that has firmness.

Chapter 11

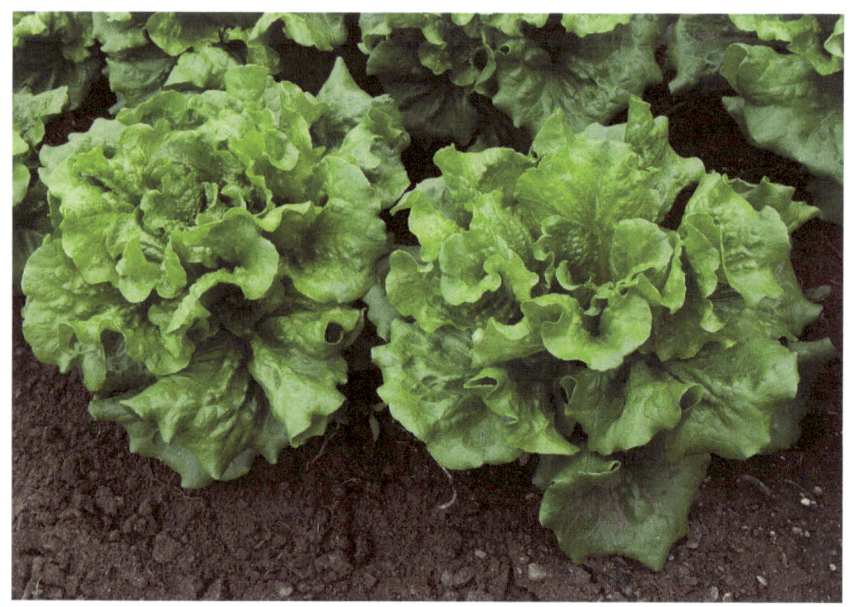

Lettuce

Lettuce are really healthy for you, it helps your digestive system it's also high in vitamin C and has a excellent value of vitamin A. when eating lettuce try to stay away from fatty dressings that add on excessive calories that are not needed for the body. Eat it natural so you can get the best results. This vegetable is almost in every dish most people that are having problems with their health in different areas eat lettuce to reduce illness or they eat them for dietary purposes. The fact remains it's a better food for the body, rich in fiber it contains potassium also phosphorus. It has been told that eating this vegetable can reduce the age related macular degeneration found in eye vision. Eating lettuces can help an individual manage weight maintenance. You can have a nutritious low calorie salad for lunch or dinner. Also after completing jogging, aerobics, pull ups, bench pressing sessions. Make sure the lettuces are clean check for the darker green lettuces it contains the right amount of beta-carotene.

You can store them in a container or plastic wrap ready to be place in the refrigerator. I enjoy eating them with lots of different fruits for a flavorful sweet taste.

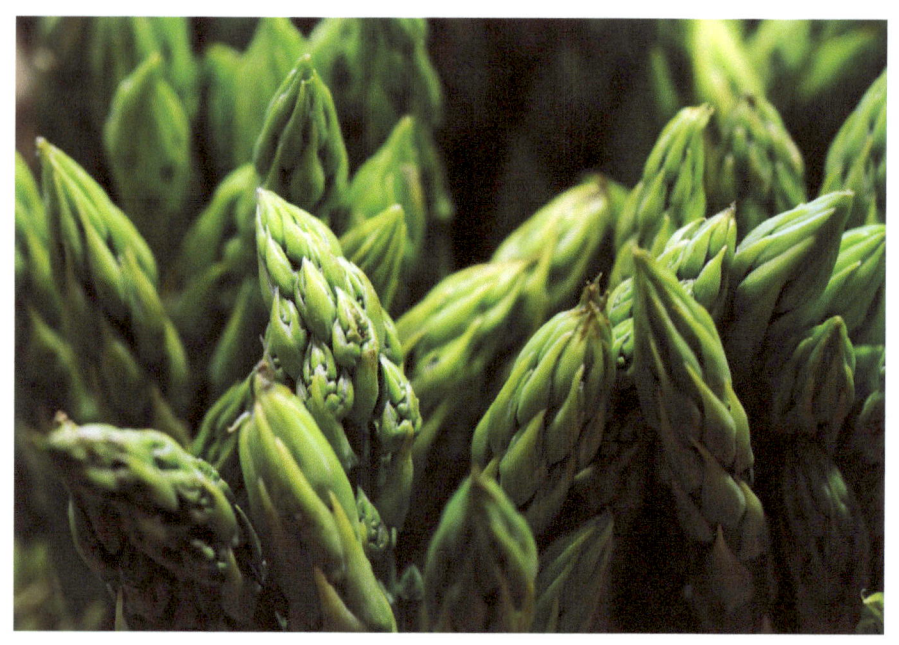

Asparagus

Asparagus come in three colors purple, white or green they are members of the lily family. It's produced in different countries like Mexico, North America, China. They are a excellent source containing Folic acid that has the ability to control homocysteine which is a factor for heart disease, lowering cancer risk and cognitive dysfunction. It contains vitamin B plus vitamin C which can strengthen blood cells also protect towards oxidative damage. Asparagus has a substance that's called protodioscin which can aid against and reduce bone loss. It also has the ability to enhance sexual desire and erection growth. The vegetable has been used as a herbalists treatment towards toothaches, arthritis also infertility and problems dealing with swelling known as rheumatism. Most people eat asparagus in different ways some eat them raw after washing them thoroughly with water others grill them and some people fry it. The best way I think would be more beneficial eating them raw and eat the organic asparagus. Make sure they are compact. Green firm tips.

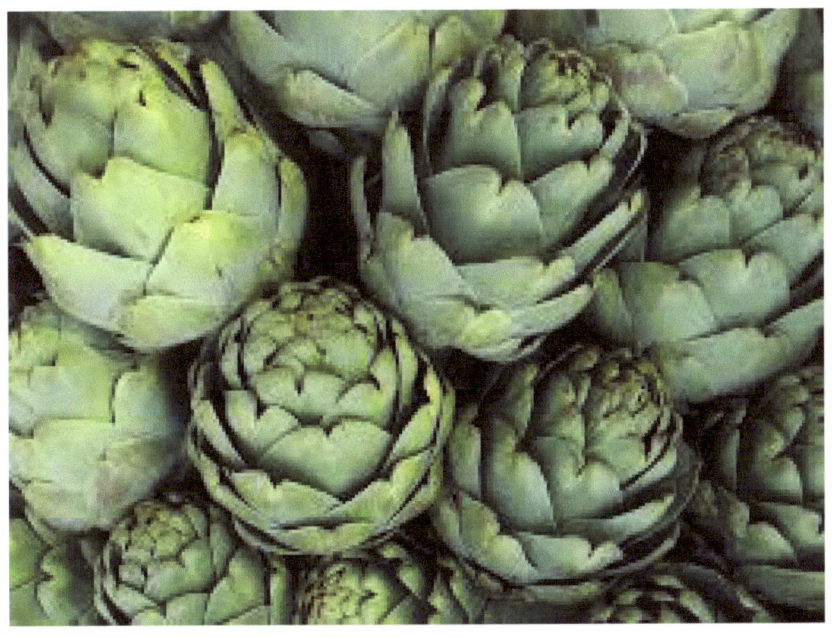

Artichokes

Artichokes can come in different colors from light green to very dark purple this vegetable has been known to help in various situations towards healing process involving individual biological system. It has a great source of vitamin C contains fiber which is good for dietary purposes. It has potassium also magnesium. Artichokes has a substance which can support and protect liver and heart disease by preventing cholesterol build up that is very harmful for the body. It has been known to relieve stomach pains as well cleaning the blood in ways of detoxifying the body gall bladder and liver. Some people have used it as a treatment for snakebites, itching and anemia. Artichoke has the ability to restore sufficient flow to the veins and arteries.

Always wash the artichokes well make sure to remove decompose leaves. Some people cook them by steaming them or boiling them. Whatever way makes you happy to prepare this delicious vegetable. When you're outside grocery shopping select the one's that feel heavy with tight leaves, dark purple or dark green colors.

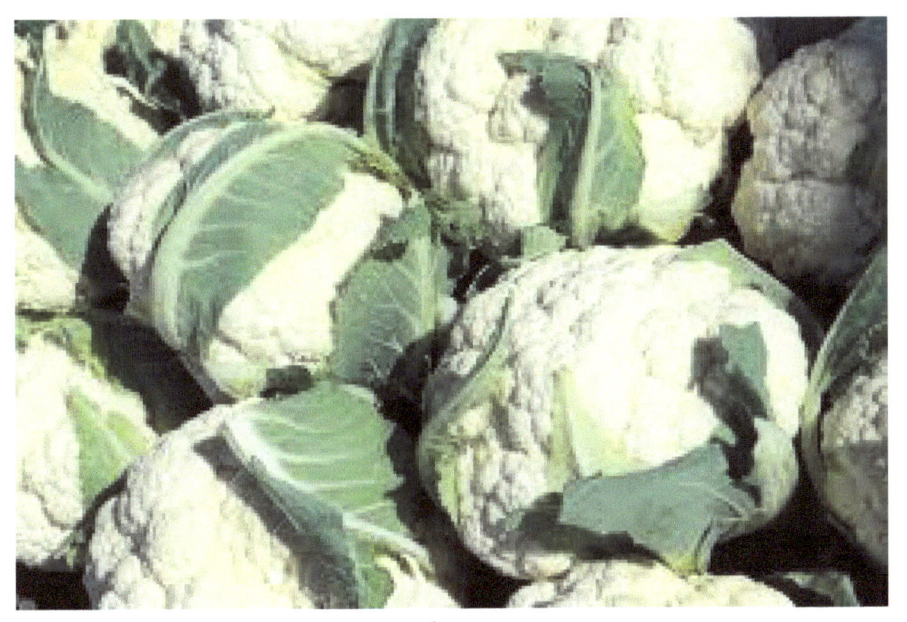

Cauliflower

Cauliflower which comes in several colors white, light green and purple but among them all white is the most common variety color found. Cauliflower has a great substance of vitamin C, vitamin B which contains Folate plus biotin. It also contains Sulforaphane which produce liver enzymes that blocks cancer evolving chemicals preventing them from damaging the vessel. This great vegetable can help in many ways by stopping lung cancer cells from forming. It has the ability to stop the growth of prostate cancer. The vegetable can decrease rheumatoid arthritis. You can eat cauliflower raw with dipping sauce some people cook them in their soups. It can also be put in casseroles and quiche. When you are at the supermarket picking out the best cauliflower make sure it looks white with creamy colors on the heads.

It should hold firm as well compact when you lift them they should be heavy.

Chapter 12

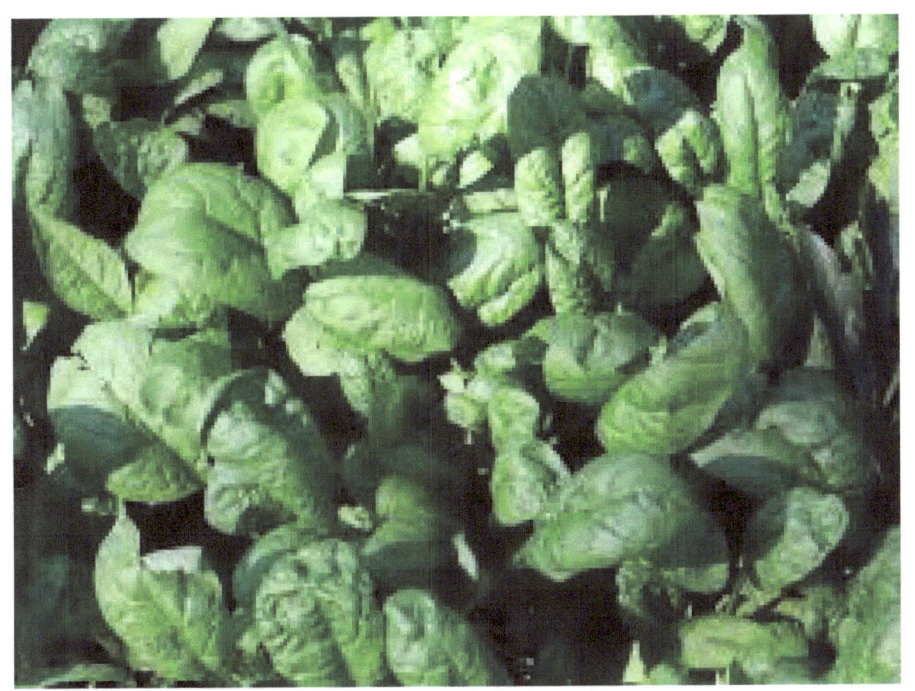

Spinach

Spinach is very nutritious and delicious it contains a great source of vitamin K and is high in fiber. It has many great minerals known as iron, magnesium and calcium also manganese which are all excellent protein for the body. Spinach contains a high amount of vitamin A which can give protection to our beautiful eyes. These compounds keep your vision healthy zeaxanthin also carotenoids and lutein. Eating spinach every three days can relieve symptoms of depression and neuritis. It can also reduce macular degeneration significantly by lowering the risk factors in ageing. Other than some vegetable spinach contains the greatest amount of

anti-proliferative. Some people boil their spinach and add a little butter and veggie herbs. Some people make delicious smoothies. I like to put it in wheat croissant bread with a sprinkle of garlic. It's not good to eat spinach from a can, can vegetable are unhealthy for you because it contains chemical that can be very bad for the heart. This vegetable has the ability to lower the occurrence of developing cataracts it's also known to increase brain function where tissue has been damaged.

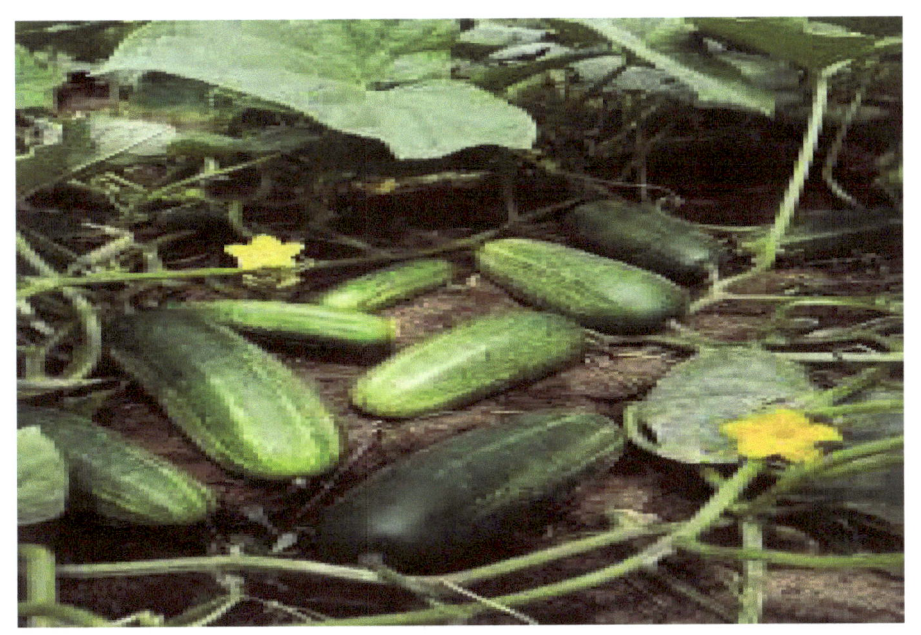

Cucumber

Cucumber they come in a dark rich green color mouth watering tasty and very healthy for the body. There good for salad dishes or eating them with vinegar. Also eat them raw peeling off the outer green skin, they are very rich in water content as well contain diuretic and anti-inflammatory which aids in dissolving uric acid which works excellent for the long jeopardy of health on the intestinal track. It has been known that the cucumber juice can be used on the outer skin of the body which will reduce inflammation of the skin also hydrates by protecting it. When purchasing the cucumber make sure you pick the organic farm produced ones make sure its unwaxed cucumbers. This vegetable contributes to the eyes also skin rehabilitation it contains vitamin C plus A. Also contains proteins known as calcium and iron. The antioxidant is very important in the related issue above. Containing vitamin K, fiber, beta carotene makes the cucumber very nutritious in minerals.

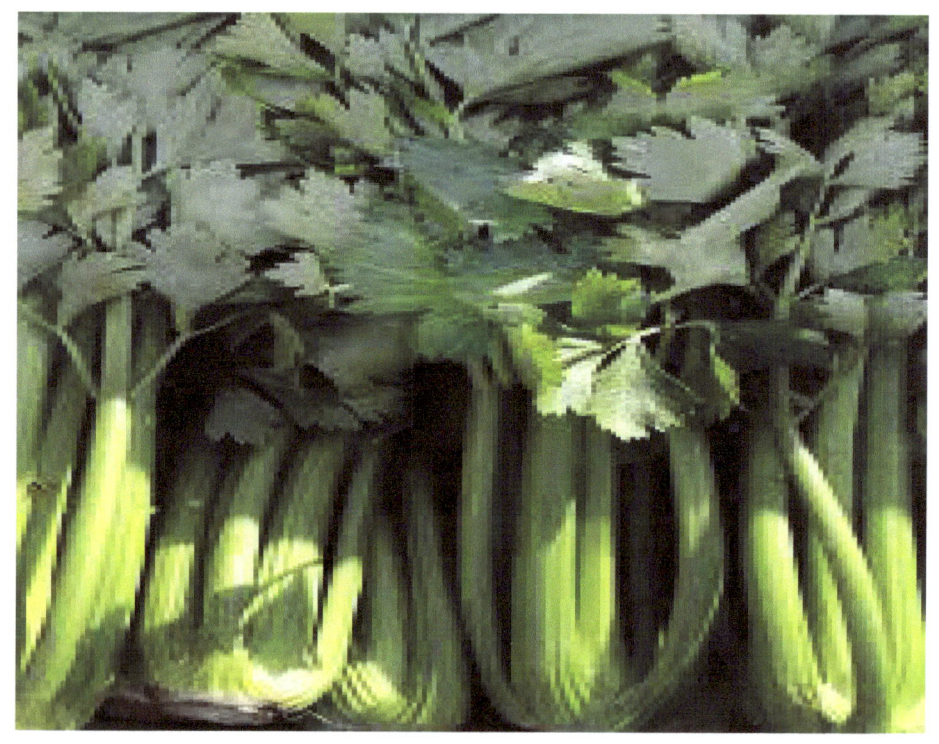

Celery

Celery this important fresh vegetable contains many minerals vitamin K which develop bone mass which will promote the activity that's called osteotrophic, It's located in the bone. It also has been used in Alzheimer's disease it has the ability to limit neuronal damage inside the brain. Celery contains a substance called coumarin which helps enhance activity that relates to white blood cells. It has been said that celery can lower blood pressure and lower cholesterol. It has been known to treat migraine headaches plus muscle pains. Most restaurants that you know serve this wonderful vegetable as a side dish. It can come chopped up on a plate with different kind of dips to place them in different sources for tast, use veggie dip it's more healthy and natural for the body intake system. Celery has a rich light and green color it will help your immune system become stronger.

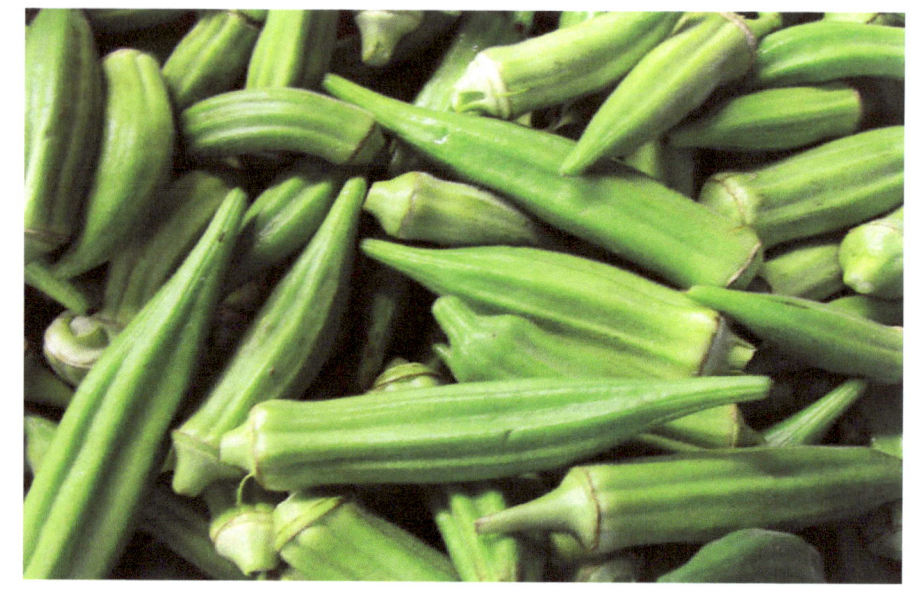

Okra

Okra which is very low in calories among the vegetable family they are a great substance to dietary fiber. These minerals plus vitamins can control build up of cholesterol plus help with weight reduction solution. The mucilaginous that's contained in the okra can help relax the flow in the peristalsis when digesting food particles by relieving

the condition in constipation, it's very high in vitamin A which is healthy pertaining to xanthin also lutein and beta carotenes. This green vegetable has a high source in levels of antioxidants which will maintain mucus membranes plus help the skin condition. This natural vegetable can protect lungs as well as oral cavity cancer. It has the ability with the substance called folates to decrease incidence pertaining to neural tube defect which is cause in offspring. The vitamin C contained in the okra can develop immunity which will act against infections by getting rid of the cough also cold. Vitamin K in okra works against clotting enzymes. You can cook okra in tomatoes sauce or even in garlic sauce giving it a good tasty flavor. You can also roast them just a little bit the way you want thanks for all the nutrients that this wonderful vegetable can provide. You can steam it lots of people cook it differently like the Mexicans, Japanese and Dominicans.

Chapter 13

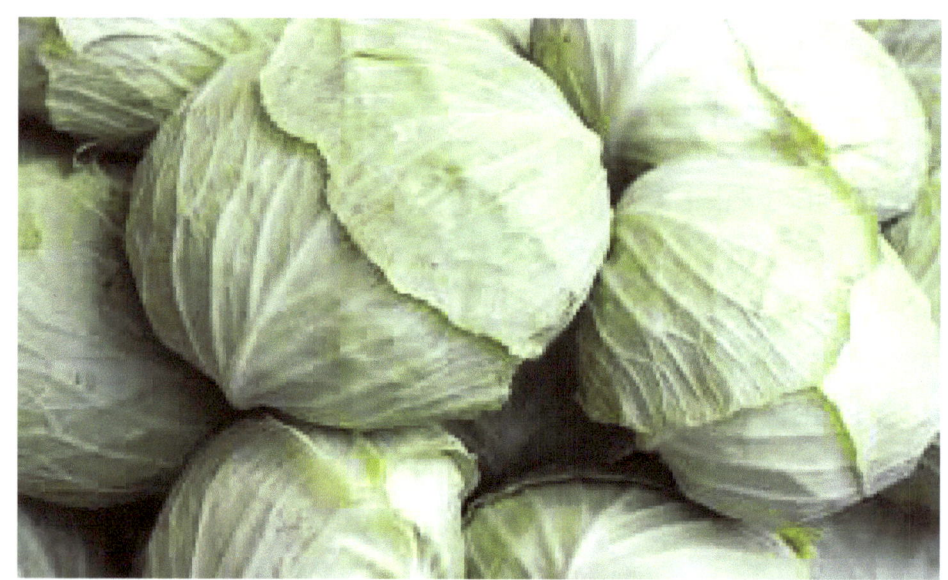

Cabbage

Cabbage white heads are very good for you in health it has an incredible source of nutrients that are excellent for the body. Let me introduce them isothiocyanates , zea-xanthin, lutein, and indole-3-carbinol these wonderful minerals work towards protecting the colon also the breasts and prostate cancer by reducing the LDL which is cholesterol bad levels in the blood. The vitamin C works against harmful infection by freeing radicals. It has a great source of vitamins known as pantothenic acid and pyridoxine, thiamin which will help in replenishing the body needs. Cabbage contains other minerals like iron, potassium, as well magnesium and manganese which contribute to maintaining blood pressure and the heart rate. The vitamin K in the cabbage white heads can promote osteotrophic that's and activity in the bone metabolism. Most of us appreciate cabbage a long side different dishes with a little seasoning dressing. Make sure the sodium is very low on the seasoning dressing to provide better health.

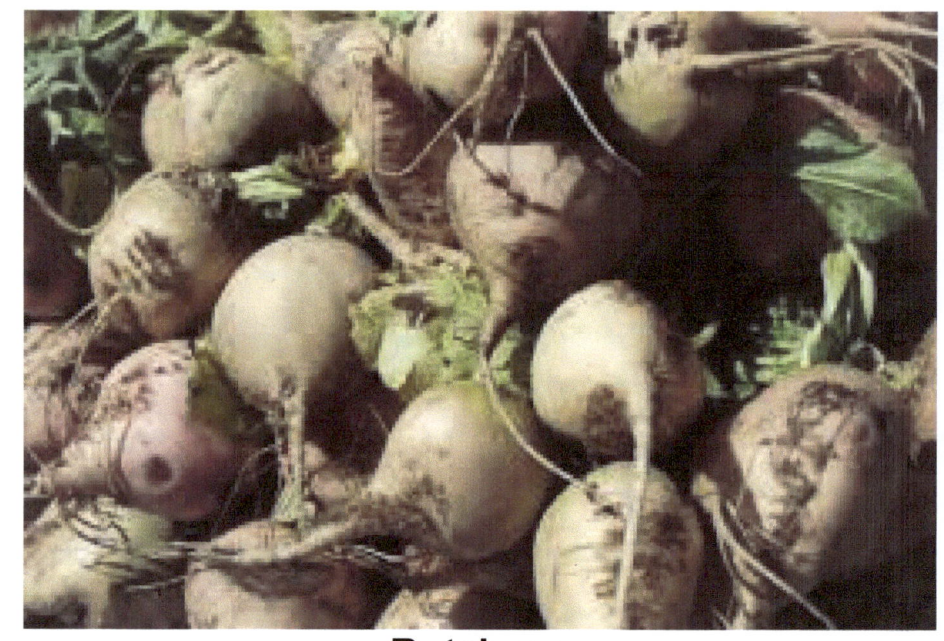

Rutabaga

Rutabaga has a great source of antioxidant nutrients and vitamin C it also has powerful anti-inflammatory which has the ability to minimize wheezing in people who are suffering from asthma. It works well with the digestive system by increasing stamina. It has the ability to balance blood sugar plus decrease cardiovascular disease. Rutabaga contains vitamin A which lowers cataract formation. This vegetable can minimize chances of heart stroke also decrease high blood pressure in the body as well provide proteins for nerve function. It can aid carbohydrate metabolism plus help muscle contraction. Rutabaga contains vitamin E that helps many areas of the body including the skin. It also can prevent baldness, and lessen type 2 diabetes by decreasing the sugar levels. Vegetables can keep us living for a very long time if we can appreciate them better and look at the knowledge of it's value towards the biological body. By mashing the rutabaga and adding some butter on them with sour cream they are ready to eat. You can also roast them however you like to cook them. A very delicious vegetable, that you will enjoy and receive nutritious proteins.

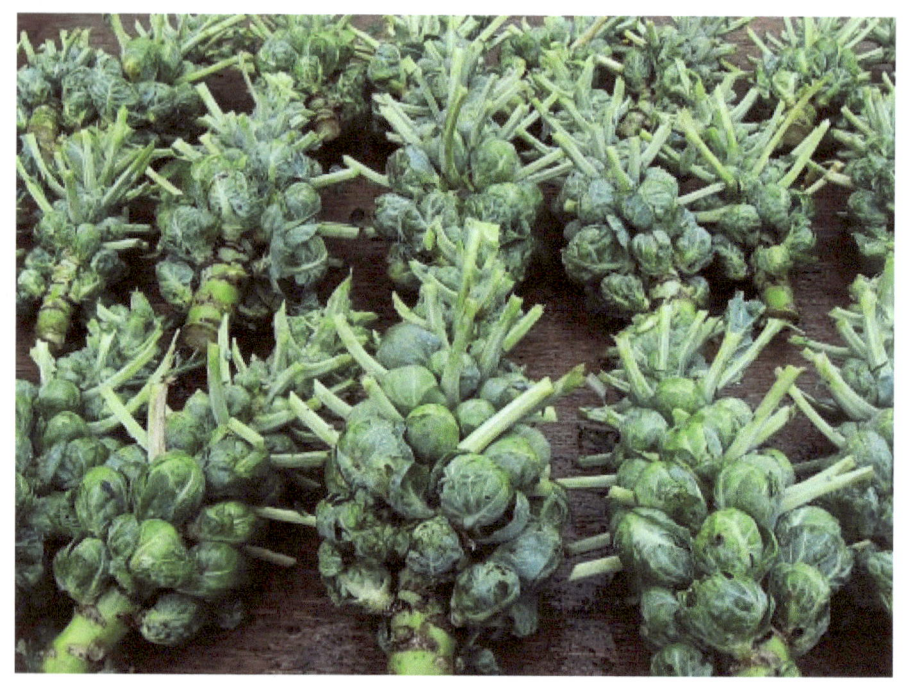

Brussels sprouts

Brussels sprouts are very healthy in many ways it is also a weight reduction vegetable that contain proteins relating to thiocyanates. These and more vegetables can offer protection to common known areas that can be affected on the colon causing prostate cancer. This vegetable has a substance in it called sinigrin and glucoside which aids against colon cancer. The zea-xanthin in the Brussels sprouts provide protection from UV rays by the sun filtering the light that is absorbed in the eyes which will prevent retinal lost. It also has the ability to help elderly people that have macular degeneration disease. Brussels sprouts are very high in vitamin K which contributes to bone health. When you buy Brussels sprouts make sure they are fresh, when you take them home wash them clean and remove any damage discolored leaves. It would be wise to soak the Brussels sprouts in salt water to remove insect eggs also dust particles. Never over cook this vegetable, five minutes would be recommended we need all the minerals it provide for health purposes.

Chapter 14

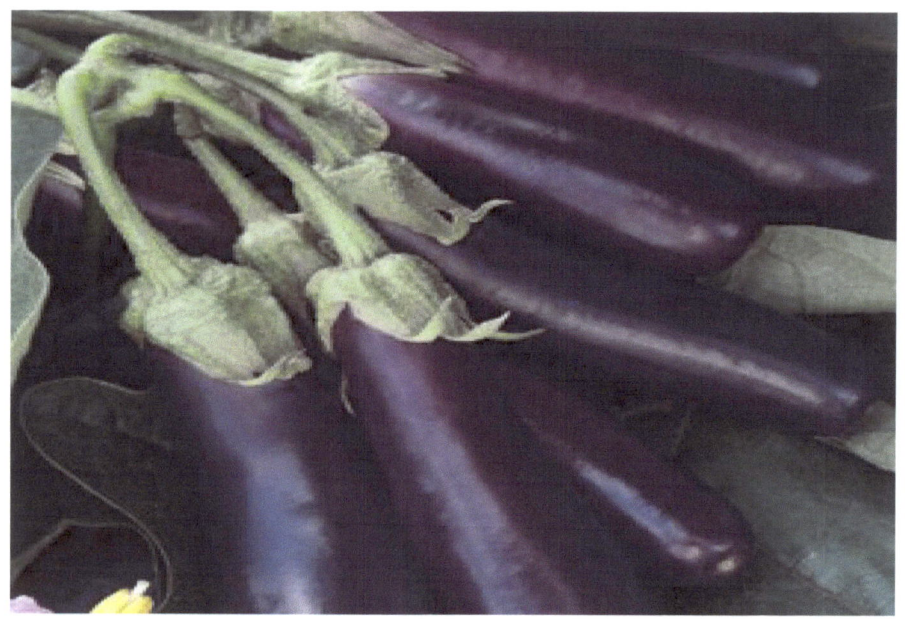

Eggplant

Eggplant this outstanding vegetable can be effective toward the balance of high blood cholesterol by controlling it. Eggplants contain a substance called anthocyancins which has the potential to work against inflammation and aging, also neurological diseases. The skin of the eggplant comes in different colors purple or dark blue. It contains many vitamins plus minerals like pyridoxine, thiamin and niacin.

These are all vitamin B proteins that are needed. The potassium in the eggplant can aid against hypertension which will benefit the blood and body function. When purchasing eggplant make sure it's firm and shiny. Must be solid avoid old stock. Always wash your vegetable to remove all outside harmful things. Add salt to clean. You can eat eggplant in many ways some people apply it in their salads, some even bake it and cook it with garlic tomatoes sauce and parmesan. Grilled eggplants are very good. Preparing this great vegetable that comes with many recipes. Create your own technique which is suitable for you. Enjoy this healthy treat.

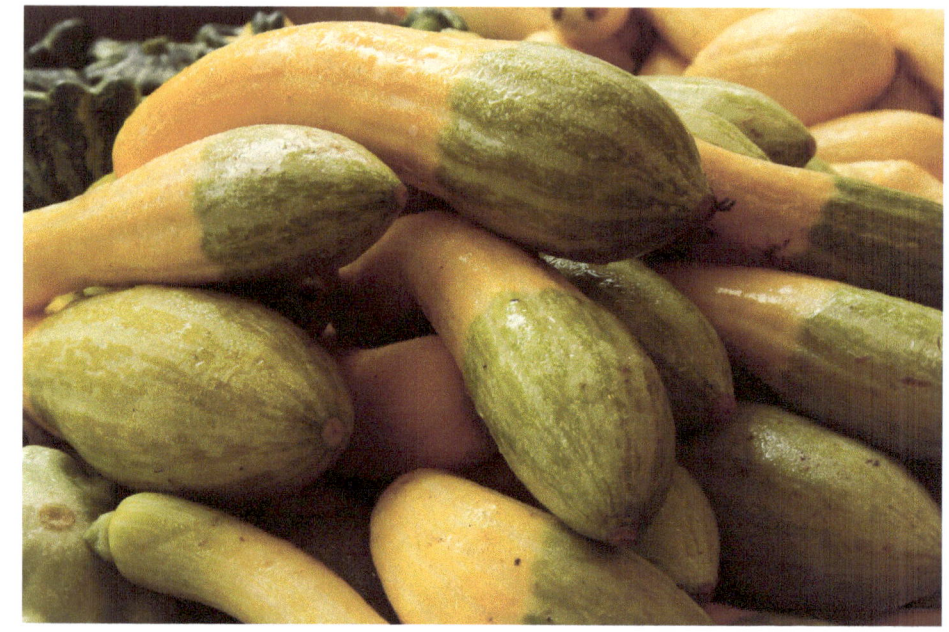

Squash

Squash contains phosphorus, riboflavin, folate, bet-carotene and fiber. The potassium in the squash relates to the electrolyte that aid in balancing body fluids. The manganese substances in the squash provide aid in processing fat. This vegetable has been known to reduce heart diseases, strokes by decreasing fat and lowering cholesterol. I enjoy when the righteous brothers and sisters bake and sale squash pies, they do not put white sugar in it they put brown sugar and butter which is healthier for the body. All the items that are used are natural from the farm thanks to the brothers and sisters for this wonderful squash pie and the navy bean pie. The minerals in both squash and navy bean can prolong life.

It has the ability to remove unwanted toxins that are in the body. It can help against prostate and colon cancer, and aid our beautiful vision. It also helps the bones by providing nutrients we need. Eating this vegetable will benefit you in all kinds of ways towards your health. This great vegetable would be my number one dish squash.

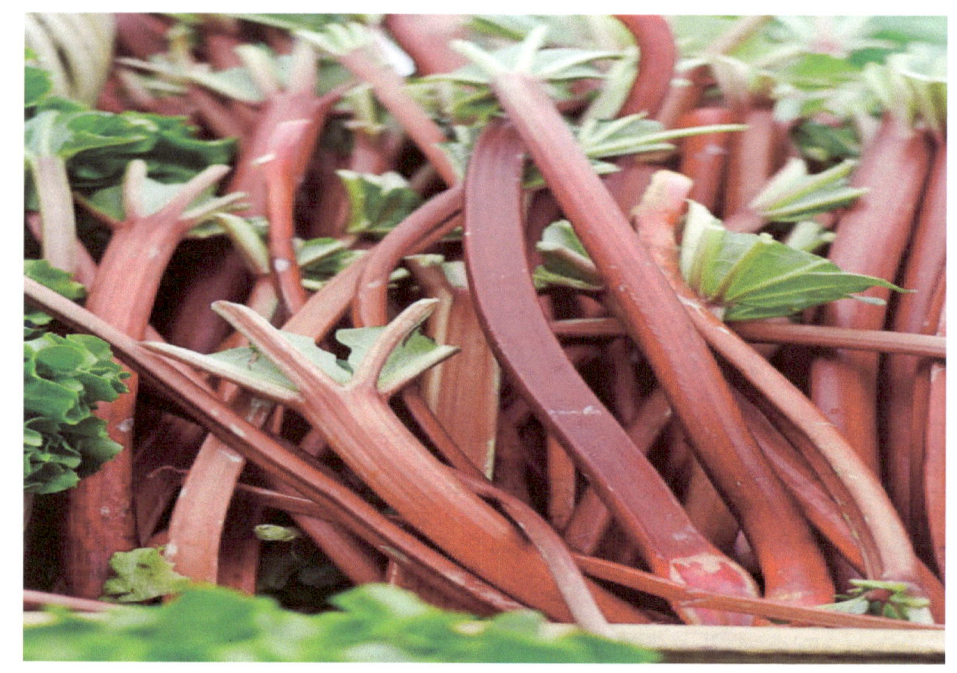

Rhubarb

Rhubarb contains vitamin B six also thiamin and niacin. The vitamin A in rhubarb has a very strong substance pertaining to anti-oxidant which is required by the physical body. It aids in maintaining the mucus membranes as well the skin our largest organ in the human body. The stalks also on the rhubarb have very high levels of protein which contains different minerals phosphorus and copper as well iron plus calcium let's not forget potassium. The vitamin K helps in maintaining the role in potential bone strengthening promoting osteotrophic that works on the formation of the bone. Rhubarb is very rich in vitamin B known as thiamin. When you are out buying rhubarb from the supermarket buy it fresh, make sure the stalks are shinning bright red firm avoid slump hang over dull ones. It's a good vegetable for many things jellies and jams different sauces and tarts also muffins as well pancakes. This is a great vegetable of many uses.

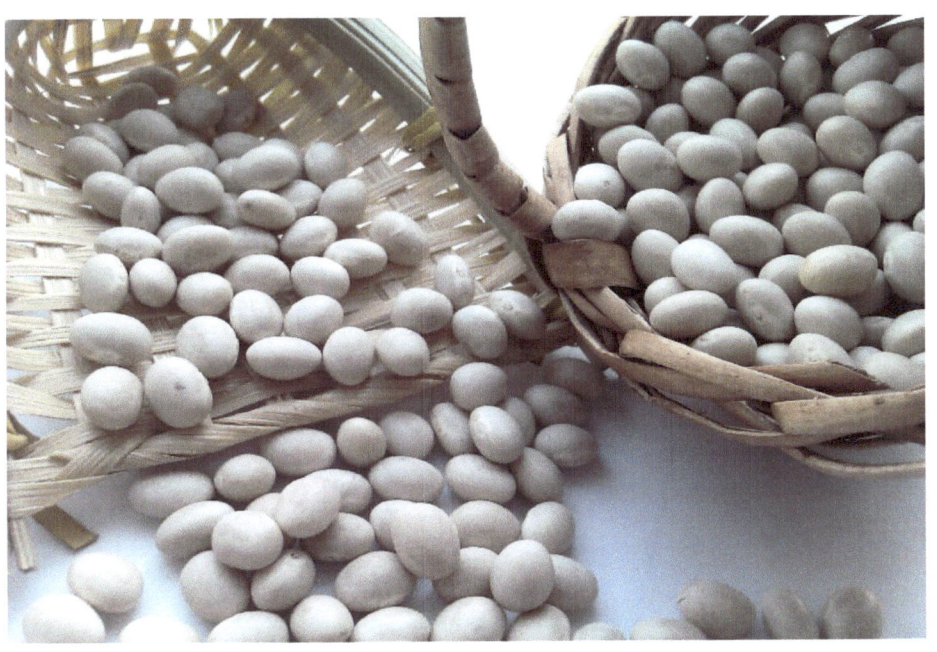

Navy beans

Navy bean let me start by saying this navy bean has a lot of importance to the total physical body it can maintain the entire body by feeding the brain, muscles, blood, liver, heart, arteries, lungs, and the nervous system. It has all the nutritional elements that are provided for the whole system of the body. It is excellent in lowering cholesterol. The high fiber in it prevents blood sugar levels from rising people with diabetes should make this vegetable their number one food on the list navy beans are fat free quality protein that contain many great sources of nutrition vitamin B1 and maganese as well folate and these minerals phosphorus and magnesium let's not forget iron and copper if you are having digestive disorder the navy bean can help relieve the problem at hand the navy bean can lower heart attack risk also the navy beans can reduce radiation in the body caused by cell phone ,television ,radio there are more on the list that can activate cancer cells. It's good cooking navy bean pie ,soups and a lot more delicious healthy dishes.

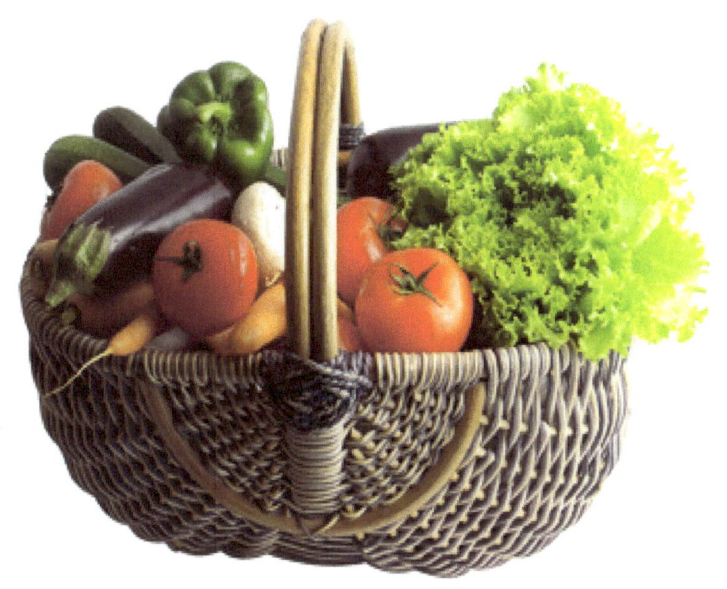

This book is recommended for children, women, men's health the wellness of oneself fitness will be whatever exercise you choose with care and balance jog, run, pushups, pull-ups, sit ups, jumping jacks, aerobics, weight lifting, walking, Football, baseball, basketball, bowling. I know there are more exercises, hobbies and sports I just mentioned a few.

In time you will find this information useful these basic steps will change our life and save money in our pockets. Remember we only live once so make the best of it while you're here you don't want to be hooked up to a machine in the hospital for your last days on the earth. Enjoy life and respect life! The benefits would be put that work in mentally and changes will come physically, this choice is not hard the mind is a strong tool feed it right and it will work for you. I would like to show you some exercises follow the green arrow, view the different activities.

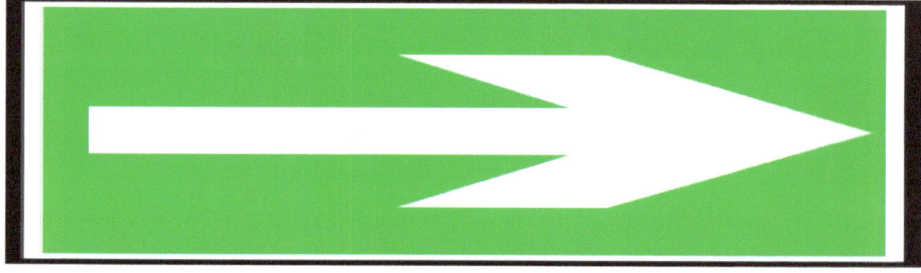

Chapter 15

Exercises

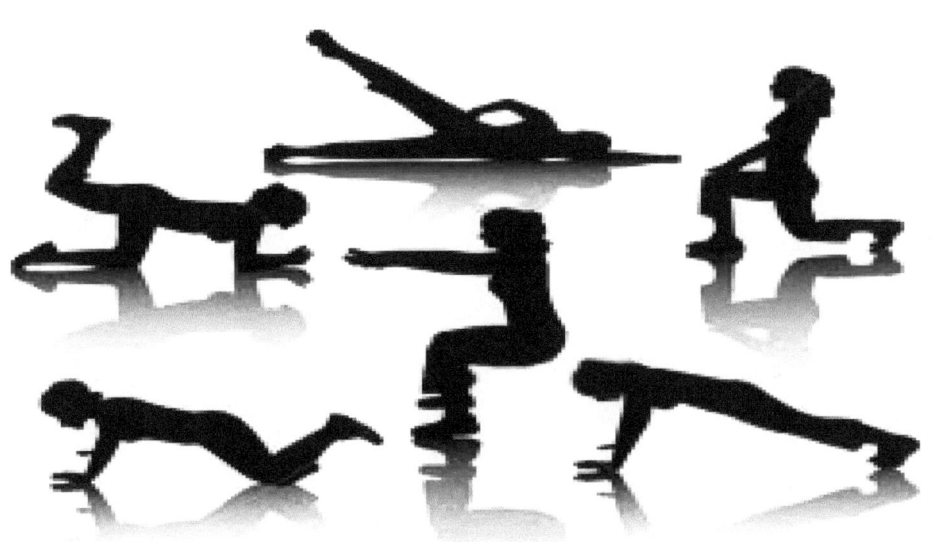

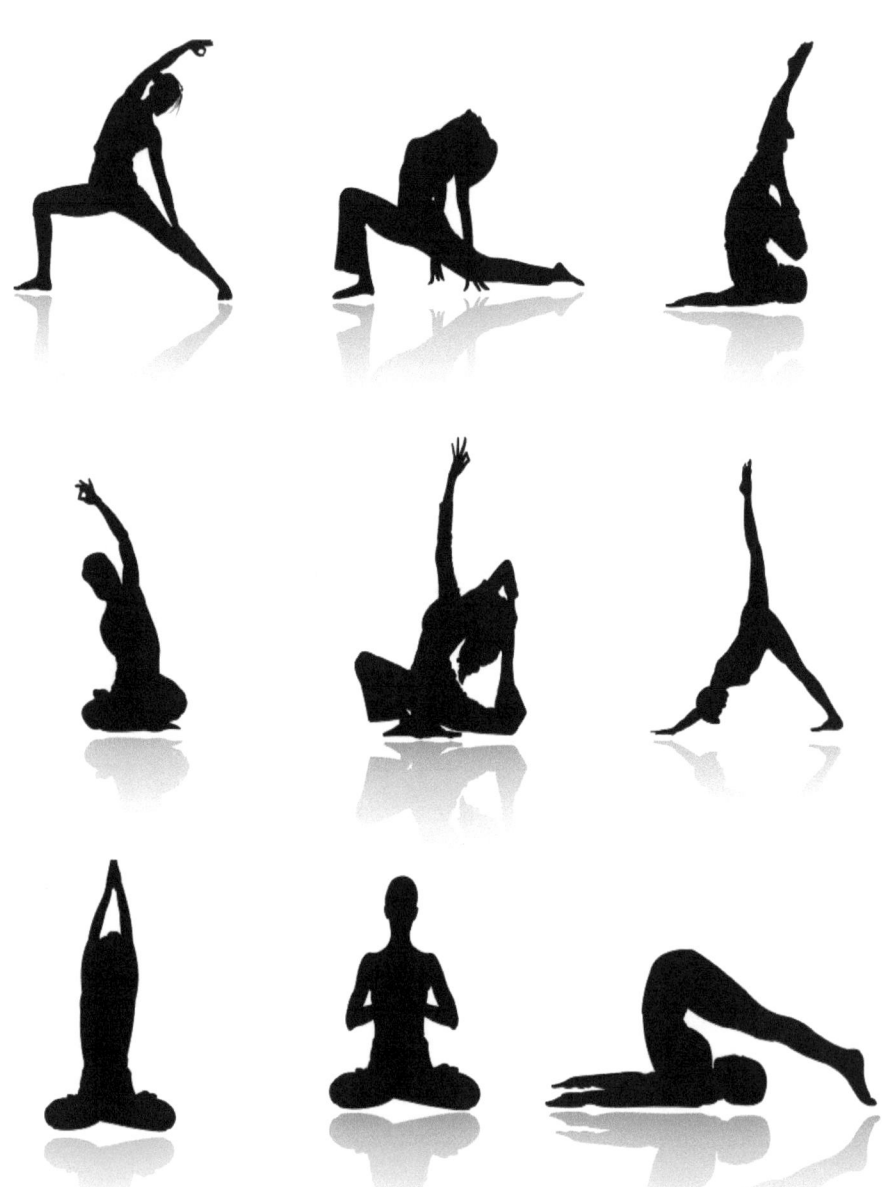

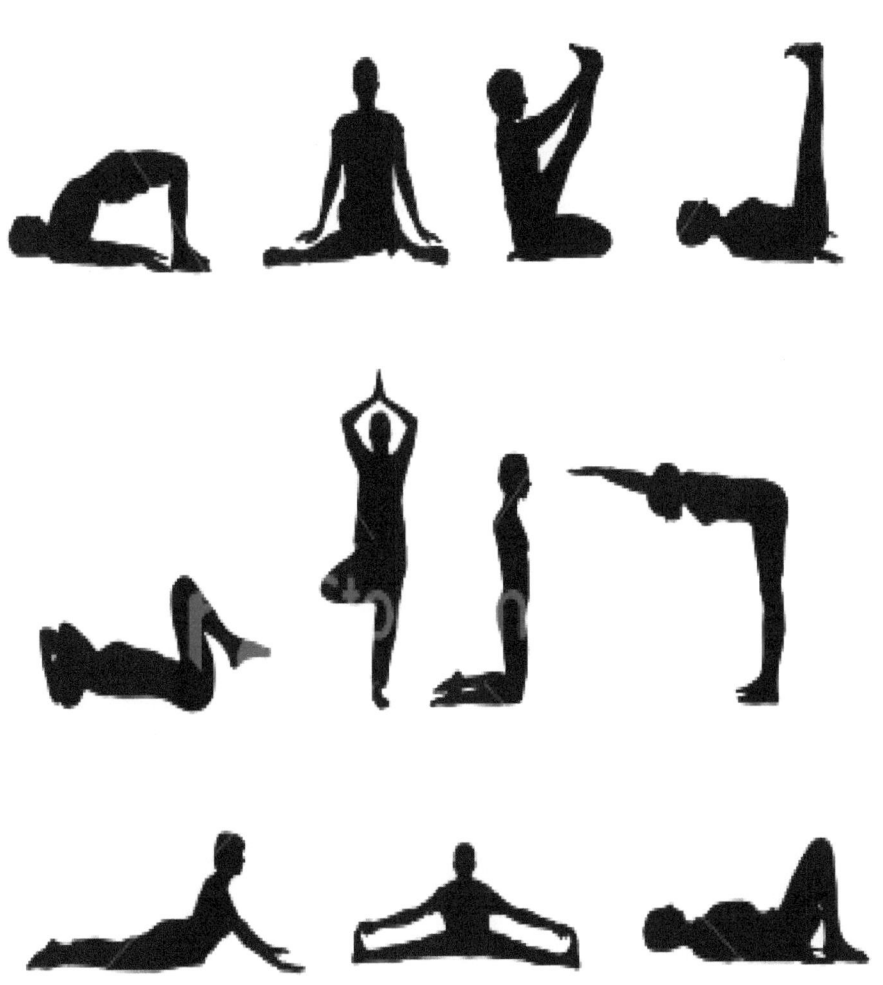

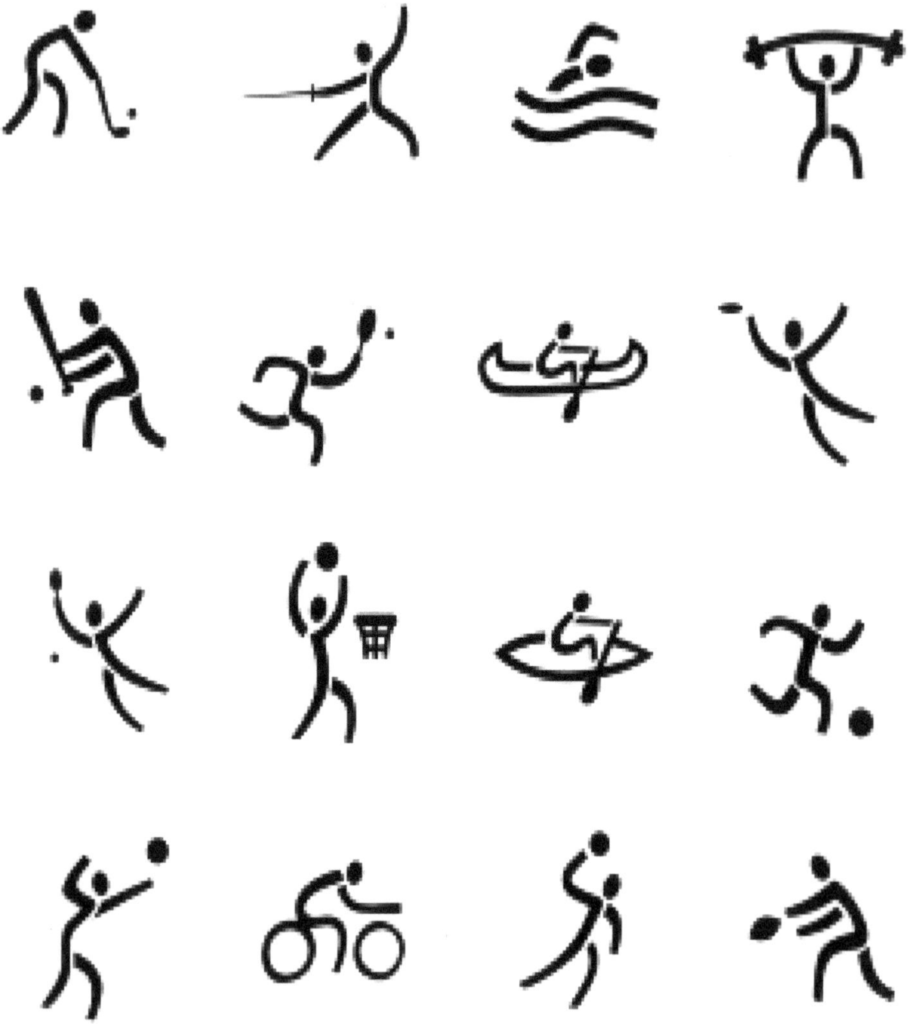

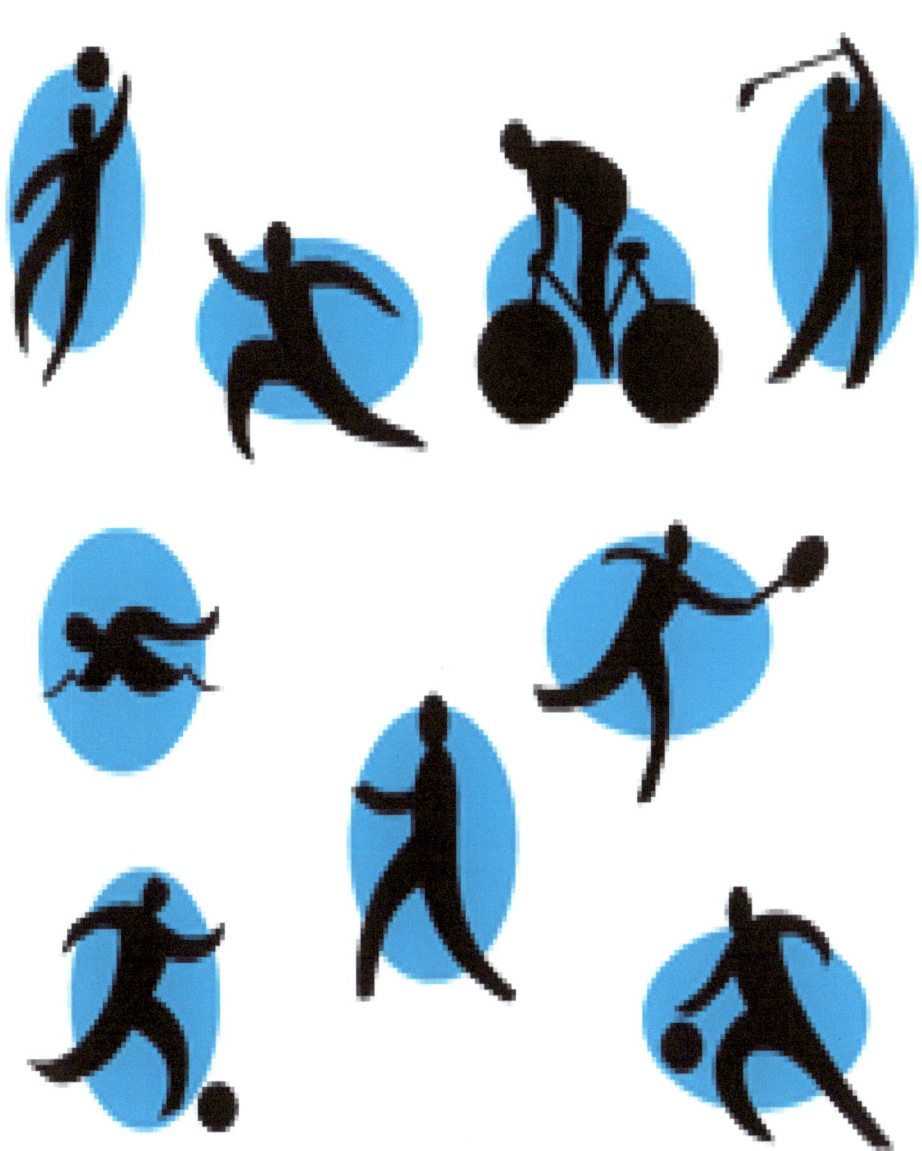

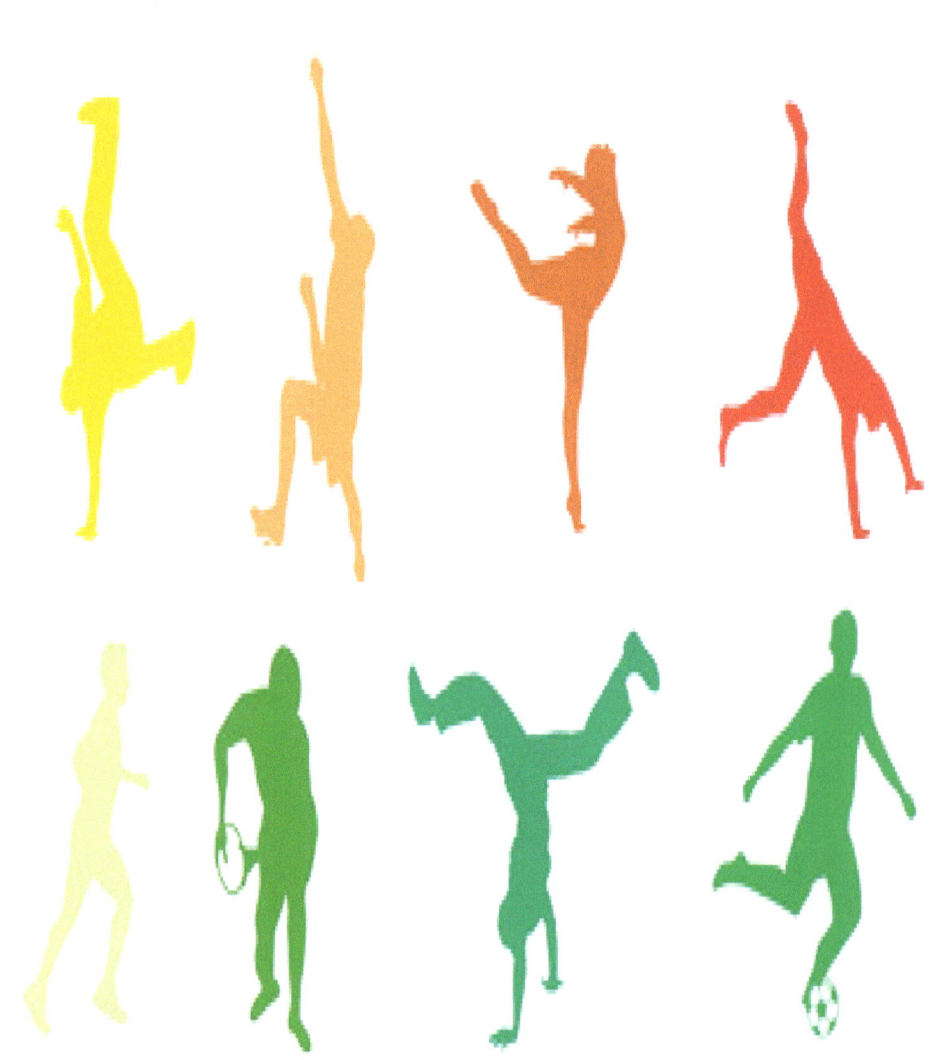

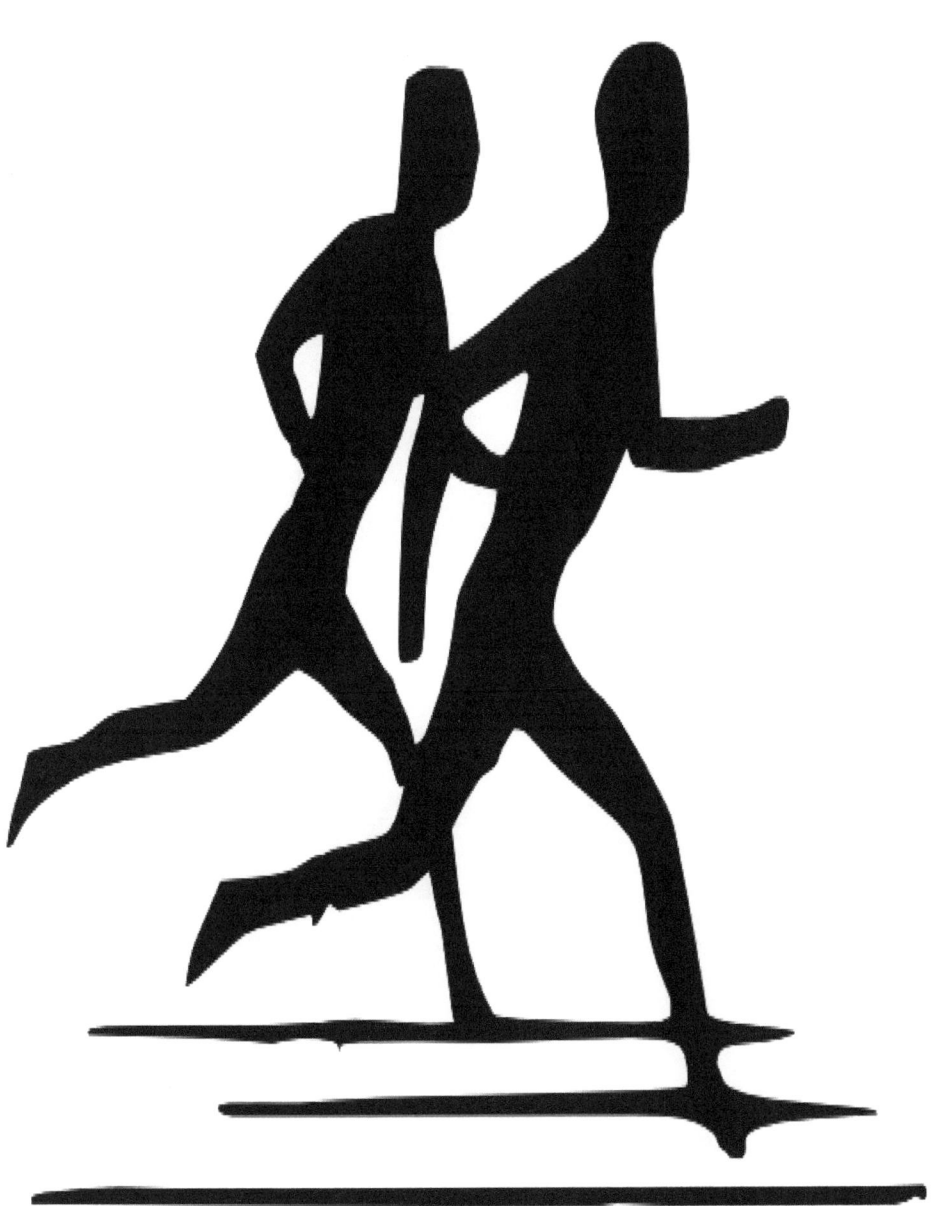

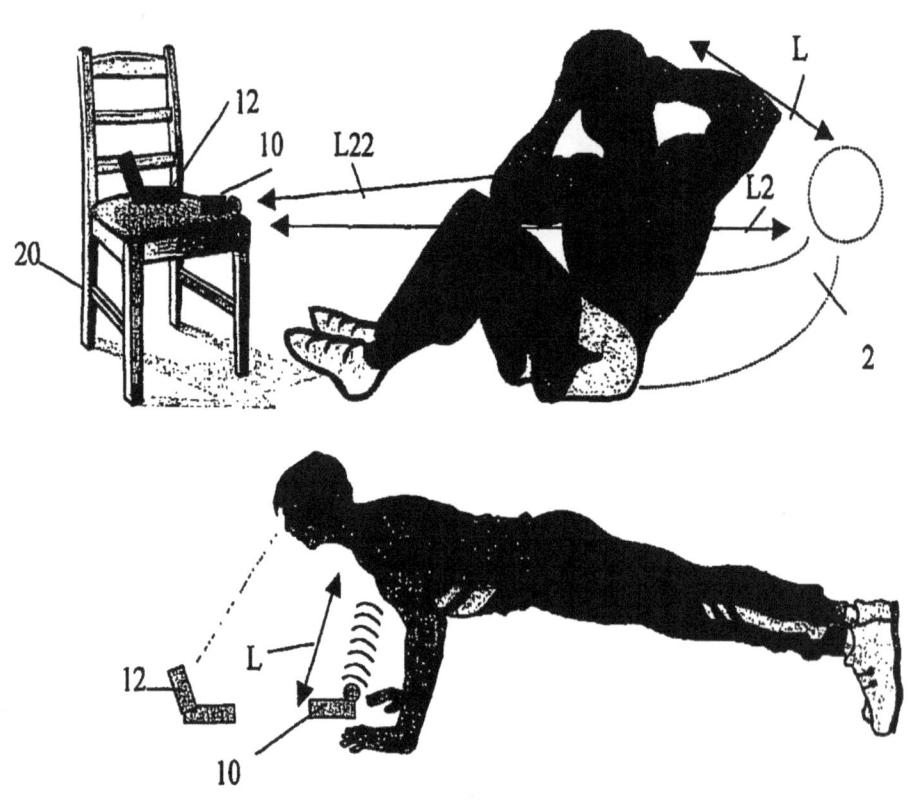

www.ingramcontent.com/pod-product-compliance
Lightning Source LLC
Chambersburg PA
CBHW050809290526
45792CB00001B/38